How to Get Rid of Acne

The Ultimate Cure Guide for How to Overcome Your Acne Forever

Table Of Contents

Introduction

This short, concise book contains proven steps and strategies on how to overcome your acne forever. These are effective ways that are clinically proven to be helpful as a cure to acne breakouts. Practicing these methods to get rid of your acne will help you in your problem and make your skin appear clearer and fresher.

We will dive into what is going on in your skin, how your skin reacts to different triggers, how your eating, drinking, and exercising habits can influence your skin, as well as what work is required of you to get past the roadblocks you have.

It is recommended that you take notes while reading this book. This will ensure that you get the most out of the information in here. The notes will help you to pinpoint exactly what you need to implement, and by writing things down, you will be able to recall specifics and how to handle certain situations when they arise.

Lastly, it is encouraged that you do your own research on the topics you want to look deeper into. We must be aware of what is true and false regarding skin care, or else we become susceptible to falling for scam products like some of the creams and lotions out there which promise instant results.

The more you understand about your own body and its triggers, the better off you'll be. To overcome an acne problem, it will take some work on your part but you can do it! So remember to read with confidence and an open mind!

Chapter 1:

Oh No! Acne!

How would you feel if when you woke up in the morning, the first thing that you saw when you looked in the mirror was a big, red, round mark on your forehead? That would be so annoying, right? For some people acne break outs are so frequent that this becomes a regular occurrence for them.

Acne ruins not only your face but sometimes your day as well. For most people who suffer from acne issues, they don't have to worry about any serious health risks. However, it can damage one's self-esteem in today's world, which is very looks-conscious.

Today's technology has developed a lot of clinically proven ways to treat acne effectively. However, there is just one problem with this—money. Not all can afford such effective and exclusive treatment modalities. Yet, there are practical and natural ways that can still help solve or reduce your problems.

Acne is a skin problem that affects all kinds of people at all ages. However, mostly teenagers and young adults are the ones who suffer from the serious self-esteem issues that acne can bring about. Why is this so? A combination of factors. Firstly, teenagers and young adults are dealing with so many hormonal changes in an extremely short period of time. Secondly, they are more active than their older and younger counterparts and often times they haven't adopted proper hygienic habits, or aren't as educated on the subject.

There are certainly factors that contribute to the appearance of acne such as dirt, stress, lack of sleep, improper diet, vices, oily skin, and genetics. Another is because of an effect in the hormones that is common to teenagers undergoing changes in their bodies.

There are also certain conditions that can worsen acne, and they are as follows:

Rosacea

Over 16 million people in the U.S.A. are affected by Rosacea, a skin disorder that brings forth small, red, and pus-filled bumps on the skin, the forehead, and the cheeks. The problem with this is that there is no known cure for it, and it has its own set of symptoms that may even worsen acne.

Adrenal Cortical Carcinoma

This is a rare disease that involves a cancerous growth in your body, mostly on the adrenal glands that are found on top of your kidneys. The adrenal cortex produces androgens and cortisol, and when there is an excessive production of these hormones, the body is not able to handle it, and thus, pimples and acne appear.

Polycystic Ovarian Syndrome (PCOS)

In this condition, a woman's progesterone and estrogen hormone production are messed up.

PCOS affects a person's appearance, in a way that brings forth acne, Not only that, PCOS also affects cardiac function, menstrual cycles, and a person's fertility as well. It affects 1 in 10 to 20 women of childbearing age.

Cushing Syndrome

When you have abnormally high levels of cortisol in your body, which becomes a problem when you use corticosteroid medications too much, your cortisol levels begin to act up and give you acne, or other skin problems. Aside from acne, skin healing also becomes much slower because of this condition.

Excessive Sweating

Excessive sweating is actually a medical problem that has different triggers, and in some instances it is hard to decipher what actually caused the problem. This can also be a syndrome of hyperthyroidism or menopause, and is suffered by at least 3 percent of Americans. The problem is that people think it's just a trivial matter, and thus, they do not seek treatment, causing the condition to worsen.

Unwanted or Excessive Hair in Women

Excessive hair can be truly irritating, and can cause pimples, acne, or other skin irritations.

Premenstrual Syndrome (PMS)

This happens at least 5 to 11 days before a woman's monthly period, and at this point, a woman may be highly emotional or irritable, and because of that, acne becomes prevalent. This is mostly a risk for women who are suffering from mood disorders such as depression, and who have family histories of PMS or depression, as well.

However, these factors are easy to avoid as long as you have enough discipline to care for your body.

These natural and affordable ways of treating acne are clinically proven to be effective. Some methods do not only treat your acne but will also introduce you to a healthier lifestyle. Although these methods do not take effect right away, surely the results will last a lifetime, unlike some clinical treatments that compel you to undergo many concentrated sessions, wherein lots of time and money is wasted in the long run.

Many recommend going for the natural ways of treating a lot of diseases and conditions, not just acne problems. There are more advantages than disadvantages when going the natural route, although it does takes a little more work than using a topical cream. Nevertheless, going natural is not only affordable, but it also has minimal side effects because there are fewer chemical additives that may damage the skin. These methods can also be practiced anywhere, as everyone has access to natural treatments.

Chapter 2:

Cleansing with Water

Dirt is one cause of acne. With all the pollution around us, it is much harder to maintain cleanliness on the outside of the body, but with proper grooming, it is possible. In big cities especially, it is almost impossible to avoid the pollution in the air.

Every day, you encounter different things that cause you to acquire dirt, which contain germs and bacteria. Simply touching different surfaces outside, or even at home, can result in dirt on your body. However, simply washing your hands with water or even alcohol or hand sanitizer is enough to take care of this issue. Another key that people tend to neglect is using an exfoliating scrub in the shower. By scrubbing the pores all over your body, you go a step further in preventing dirt build up.

Many people have this habit of washing their hands before they eat, but this does not only apply here. You must also make it a habit to wash your hands before you touch your face. You'd be shocked to know how often some people touch their cheeks, nose, foreheads, and eyes throughout the day, just out of habit. If you can avoid touching these sensitive areas with dirty hands, it will greatly reduce your chance of clogging the pores with dirt.

Another simple technique to implement is to wash your face before sleeping and after you wake up. This can eliminate the dirt that has accumulated on your face throughout a busy day. It is important to wash your face often in order to remove skin impurities, dead skin cells, and extra oil in your skin. However, you should limit thorough washing of the face to two to three times a day because washing it excessively will do more harm than good. In washing your face, you should use warm water and a mild facial cleanser. Using a harsh soap can harm the skin and, in turn, cause more irritation.

Do not scrub your facial skin harshly with a washcloth, exfoliating glove or a coarse sponge; use only your hands or a very soft cloth. Always rinse your face well and dry it with a soft towel. If possible, do not use the same towel again, as a used towel can be a breeding ground for germs and bacteria.

It will only take you minimal time and effort to keep your body and face clean, but you will be able to eliminate random dirt collection in your pores by using these techniques. The truth is, if you get into the habit of doing these things everyday, you can get to the point where it only takes 5-10 minutes total each day.

Did you know that drinking water can also help prevent acne? Water does not only clean the external parts of the body but also the internal systems and organs. Doctors recommend drinking at least eight glasses of water a day to help eliminate all the unnecessary fluids in the body and ensure the proper functioning of the excretory system that is responsible for discharging wastes from the body. This is the same waste that causes unhealthy skin. We often forget that water plays a huge role in the excretion of waste through the pores. This is the same reason why many people feel much cleaner after a long, intense workout after having been stagnant for the previous months. They are essentially sweating out much of the dirt that has been trapped in their pores.

Increase your water intake to purify your outer skin as well as the inner layers. Completing the daily recommended water intake can make your skin glow and look fresh. This also helps reduce the risk of skin issues down the road. If you aren't sure whether your water intake is sufficient at the moment, begin by adding a small cup of water each day, then slowly increase your intake over the span of a few weeks. Evaluate how your energy, urine color, and skin changes through this phase.

Chapter 3:

Stress Leads to Stress

Stress is one of the major factors that can cause acne. Stressing yourself out too much does not bring you any positive effects, it will only make you emotionally, physically, and mentally unhealthy. People who are stressed out either sleep too much or do not get enough sleep; neither one is good for the body.

On the other hand, lack of sleep can make you feel grumpy. Sleep plays a big role in an individual's ability to think. When one does not have enough sleep, the person's cognitive process slows down. Sleep deprivation can also lead to a lot of health problems including heart disease, stroke, and diabetes. In contrast to oversleeping, lack of sleep can then make you gain weight. It can also make you look old and make your skin look and feel unhealthy.

Typically, individuals are recommended to get at least six to eight hours of uninterrupted sleep every night. Maintaining proper sleeping hours can make your skin feel and look much healthier. If you switch from a pattern of not getting enough sleep to getting the proper amount, you will see a notable "fresh" look to your skin.

Stress and acne breakouts are directly linked to each other. When the brain recognizes stress, it automatically releases stress hormones that help thicken the hair follicles' lining, causing blackheads or whiteheads, wherein, when bacteria gets trapped, it is how pimples are formed.

Needless to say, in order to avoid these effects of stress, one must avoid becoming stressed out. Try to let negative thoughts pass without harping on them. It is important to recognize problems in your life, but thinking about them more than a brief evaluation is no longer beneficial. "Smile out" your problems. Do not let your emotions control you; it should be the other way around. In order for you to stay fit and have the clear skin you desire, you must ensure that you take care of your mental health first and foremost.

Your mind works harmoniously with your body. How you think will help determine what you will look like. Smiling decreases the possibility of breakouts and makes you look younger. It not only helps maintain good health, but also good interactions with others.

Know the source of your stress and think of ways to avoid it. Get more sleep and engage more often in exercise and other activities that would aid you in forgetting about what is stressing you out.

Pay attention to how your skin reacts in the weeks when you are caught up in your head wondering about your problems. Many people are shocked to find out that when they relax their minds more consistently, their skin begins to clear up shortly afterwards.

Chapter 4:

Bon Appetit

Caring for the body also involves eating the right amounts and right kinds of food. It is important to maintain a balanced diet because it keeps the body physically fit and healthy. Most importantly for this book, it keeps your skin fresh.

Some of the comfort foods that many enjoy are chips, fries, pizza, candy, chocolates and ice cream, but will you still want these if you found out that they are among the main causes of acne in people? Fortunately, that is just a myth.

There is no study that has proven that these foods contribute to acne breakouts and no doctors believe in such claims either. People with oily skin have the bigger propensity for acne breakout. Thus, they think that greasy foods should be avoided.

However, there are studies showing that fries, chips, or burgers do not contribute to acne. Instead, drinking a lot of milk does. So, if you are suffering from an acne problem, try avoiding dairy and stick to foods that are high in fiber, such as fruits and vegetables.

What Not to Eat

Let's start with what you shouldn't eat. Surely, there may be times when you come in contact with these foods, but as much as possible, try to stay away from them—or eat them only in small amounts. Here are the said foods:

Sugar

Sugar is definitely related to breakouts and acne. It's really about how much sugar your body gets to intake in a day. Suppose you ate a chocolate and then drank soda, what do you think will happen? Well, chances are, your blood sugar will spike, and then you might suffer from breakouts hours later. Cut back on the sugary foods and you will potentially see a huge difference!

Cow's Milk/Dairy

According to a 2010 study, there is a high link between cow's milk and acne. Apparently, dairy can irritate follicles in the face, which can then lead to acne, and may also cause a spike in your blood sugar level, which then leads to inflammation. Sebum, or skin oils, are also produced because of cow's milk, and it can also encourage the growth of skin cells, and the blockage of pores—which makes acne imminent.

Fast Food

Fast food products are often greasy and contain high levels of oil, which bring forth inflammation and acne.

Junk Food

Just like fast food, junk foods are also typically oily and salty—and will never really help you clear up your skin.

High-Glycemic Foods

High glycemic foods raise blood sugar levels as well as insulin, because they quickly break down in the body. When that happens, more sebum will be produced, and inflammation and hormonal fluctuations may occur. Examples of high glycemic foods are cakes, cookies, potato chips, whole grains, pretzels, white rice, and cereals.

What to Eat

Green Tea

Green tea actually fights acne, as proven by a number of studies, because it contains ECGC which could reduce the size of sebaceous glands, or the glands that produce sebum, and can improve your condition in a matter of 8 weeks. Aside from drinking green tea, you can also apply cloth or tea bags dipped in green tea on acne-prone areas for at least 10 to 15 minutes multiple times per week.

Flaxseed or Fish

These foods have high amounts of Omega-3 fatty acids, which help clear skin up, and tame acne breakouts and inflammation, in general. Aside from fish and flaxseed, walnuts may also do the trick, so do keep them on your grocery list.

Probiotics

Yogurt and other probiotic-filled foods such as kombucha tea, kimchi, pickles, miso soup, micro algae, sauerkraut, and kefir can reduce inflammation in the gut, and can combat oxidative stress as well.

Vegetables and Fruits

Juicing your vegetables and fruits naturally will help you obtain beta-carotene, which is known to reduce skin oils and clear up acne in the process. Toxins in the body can also be cleared away by dark, leafy greens, as well as berries.

Many fruits and vegetables are rich in Vitamins C and E, which are beneficial to the health of your skin. Avocado contains these vitamins, which reduce skin inflammation and naturally moisturize the skin. Red grapes and their seeds also contain natural ingredients that fight acne. They contain antioxidants that treat inflammatory skin conditions and also help control the side effects of the allergic reactions that manifest in the skin.

Oysters

Oysters contain zinc, and you know what zinc does? Well, it reduces acne, of course. Aside from oysters, you can also improve your diet and get more zinc by eating veal liver, toasted wheat germ, dried watermelon seeds, squash seeds, and pumpkin seeds.

Brown Rice

Brown rice is not only a helpful tool to curb satiation, but it is also a rich source of vitamins and antioxidants. For acne, Vitamin B acts as the skin's stress fighter. It helps to regulate hormonal levels and prevent breakouts.

Nuts

For quite some time, it was thought that nuts could trigger acne breakouts, but that is simply another myth. Nuts contain vitamins and minerals that are essential for healthy skin.

Garlic

Just how effective garlic is against vampires is still a matter of debate, but against acne, there is no question. Garlic fights inflammation and kills the harmful bacteria and viruses that cause acne.

Broccoli

Another skin-friendly food is broccoli. It is a great skin-clearing food that contains vitamins and antioxidants, which really work to clear out the dirty pores in our skin.

There are top foods that are recommended to get rid of and prevent acne breakouts. These foods might not cure acne overnight, but they can usually make a difference over time. People without acne problems may not have to worry about the foods they eat causing a breakout. However, they must still watch what they eat and focus on healthy foods in regards to their mental health and well-being. It's important to keep in mind that once your skin has recovered from acne breakouts, you may start bringing foods back into your diet in small amounts - but be sure to keep track of what you've introduced back in and how it is affecting your skin!

Chapter 5:

Natural DIY Remedies Against Acne

Let's briefly cover learn more natural remedies against acne that can help you get rid of this annoying condition.

Honey and Cinnamon Mask

Cinnamon is spicy, while honey is sticky—and you know what that means? Well, it means that you'll be able to create a facial mask that has amazing anti-microbial properties that can help you mitigate or get rid of your acne.

For this, you will need to mix 1 tsp of cinnamon with 2 tbsp of honey. Rinse and pat your face dry, and then apply the mixture on your face. Leave it there for a good 10 to 15 minutes, and then pat your face dry. Use paper towels to remove excess residue on your face, if ever.

Use Apple Cider Vinegar

Apple cider vinegar, also known as ACV, has the capability to kill a lot of bacteria in mere seconds. ACV works like alkaline in such a way that it balances the PH levels of your skin, which means bacteria would find a hard time living in it. ACV is also an astringent that can drive excess oils away from your body.

For this, you will need unfiltered ACV, together with fresh water. Now, what you have to do is wash your face with fresh water. After doing so, pat your face dry, and mix 1 part vinegar with 3 parts water. Dip a cotton ball into the mixture that you have just made, and leave it on your face for at least 10 minutes, or even overnight if you can. After each session, wash your face thoroughly, and make sure to re-apply several times a day. If you feel that it dries your skin out, cut back the frequency and make use of a moisturizer.

Use Egg Whites

Egg whites are amazing—and truly affordable. You see, egg whites can easily reduce faded scars and blemishes that have been left by acne on the skin. They're also full of proteins that have the ability to fight acne, and help rebuild skin cells, while soaking up sebum or excess oil. Again, this can be a bit drying so use moisturizer afterwards, if needed.

Anyway, what you need are 2 to 3 egg whites, a washcloth, and a bowl. To use these, you first have to use water to rinse your face—and don't forget to pat it dry. Then, whisk the egg whites until they get to be frothy, and just let them sit for a few minutes before you use the mixture to cover your face. Make sure that before applying a layer over another layer, you wait for the preceding layer to dry out first—the whole mask shall dry for at least 20 minutes.

After 20 minutes, rinse the mask completely with warm water, and then use a washcloth to pat it dry before putting some moisturizer on.

Milk and Honey/Yogurt

This sweet concoction may not be the most appetizing to eat, considering it can worsen acne, but by putting it on your face, it gets to have a different, positive effect. What happens is that this mixture can soothe your irritated skin because it has fat and anti-bacterial elements that can alleviate the condition, once applied topically.

For this, you'll need full-fat milk or yogurt—just at least a teaspoon, and 1 tbsp of raw, natural honey. What you have to do now is let the milk or yogurt come to room temperature, and then mix it with 1 tbsp of raw honey. Use a cotton pad to apply the mixture, and then add another one—keep on adding until you feel the mixture setting on your skin. Allow it to sit for a good 10 to 15 minutes, and then use a washcloth to wash your mask off, and get rid of loosened, dead skin cells as well!

Use Some Papaya

Do you know why papaya is used as an ingredient for most beauty products? Well, it's mostly because it is an all natural remedy that removes excess oil and dead skin cells from your face—allowing it to be soft, and naturally smooth. It also promotes lipids, which also help you get rid of excess oil. It also contains papain, an enzyme that prevents pus from forming, and reduces inflammation as well.

For this, you'll need a fresh papaya. What you should do next is wash your face with water. After doing so, pat it dry, and mash the papaya flesh until it reaches the consistency where it can easily be applied to your face. Leave it on your face for at least 15 to 20 minutes, then use warm water for rinsing. Use a moisturizer that you know agrees with your skin type afterwards.

Tea Tree Oil

Tea tree oil is always a good home remedy, and it works great against acne too! Tea tree acts like a solvent, in such a way that it unblocks the pores and removes dead skin cells because of its high anti-bacterial properties. Make sure to dilute it before use.

You'll need a small bottle of tea tree oil, cotton balls or Q-tips, and clean water. Now wash your face with clean water and then dilute the oil by mixing it with 9 parts water. Apply to the affected areas. You can also increase the amount, granted you are comfortable with it, apply it undiluted on the skin, and then use a light moisturizer afterwards.

If you have extremely sensitive skin, you can just have this diluted with aloe vera, instead.

Orange Peel Paste

Orange Peel smells great—and can also work wonders on your skin. They can refresh the skin by replacing dead skin cells with new ones, so that bacteria and dead cells that have clogged up your pores will be gone. Aside from Vitamin C, this also has great astringent qualities that can really clean and moisturize your skin, and provide you with healthy skin cells.

For this, you will need 2 orange peels, and fresh, clean water. What you should do is rinse your face with clean water. Don't forget to pat it dry. Then, pound or grind the orange peels—whichever you prefer, until it gets pasty. Add only a little at a time, and make sure not to add too much as this will make it runny and thin—which isn't what you want. Apply to the affected areas, and let it stay there for at least 20 to 25 minutes. Use water for rinsing, pat your face dry, and moisturize after.

Banana Peel

Banana peels contain lutein, a powerful antioxidant that can reduce inflammation and swelling, and could encourage healthy cell growth by saying goodbye to inflammation and swelling—which means that discomfort, redness, and the obviousness of acne will soon follow.

You only need one banana peel for this. After eating the banana, get the peel, and rub it in a circular motion on your face. Let it sit for at least 30 minutes, rinse, and evaluate the results over the next 24 hours!

Honey and Strawberries

You may be tempted to eat these, but they're great because they're mostly used in cleansers, facial scrubs, and other beauty products because not only do they small great, they are high in salicylic acid, too, which causes the epidermis to shed unwanted cells easily, neutralize bacteria, and open up clogged pores. Pores can also be shrunk, which definitely makes way for better skin, and can encourage new cell growth as well.

For this, you will need 2 tsp of good raw honey, and 3 fresh, well-washed strawberries. What you should do is wash your face, and then go ahead and pat it dry. Mash the strawberries well, mix them with honey, and just make sure they don't get runny or over-mashed in any way. Apply the mixture to your face, and let it stay there for a good 20 minutes, and then use warm water to rinse it off completely. Put on some moisturizer if your skin easily dries out, and you can try out this routine once or twice a month.

Baking Soda

Baking soda, also known as sodium bicarbonate, is great for the skin because it can easily be swooped in, and can fight bacteria and fungus because of its incredible mild antiseptic properties that can dry excess oil up, while making sure that you get to be well-exfoliated.

For this, you'll need a box of baking soda, together with fresh water. There are two ways to make this work. One would be to mix equal parts water and baking soda together so a thick paste can be formed. In thick, circular motions, massage the paste on your face for at least 2 minutes, and then leave the mask on for around 10 to 20 minutes. Use warm water for rinsing, pat dry, and moisturize.

You can also make a scrub out of it by mixing 1/2 cup of baking soda with 1/8 cup of water, and then applying it to your face. Massage it well, and rinse after 5 to 6 minutes with warm water before moisturizing.

Steam

Steam can also be quite useful in fighting acne, mostly because it opens up the pores and flushes dirt out—even those that lurk deep within the skin. You can choose to steam alone, or moisturize afterwards, but the important thing is that you have 1 pot of boiling water, 1 towel, and a large bowl with you.

Now, what you have to do is boil some water in the said pot, and then pour the contents in a large bowl after boiling. Let it cool for a few minutes, and then once it's cooled a bit, go and put your face above the bowl with towel draped over it. Take the towel off and pat your face dry after a good 10 to 15 minutes. Do this at least once or twice a day if you want to test this method out.

Lemon Juice

Lemon has natural astringent properties that is good for all skin types—definitely a plus factor—and can help you get rid of or mitigate breakouts. Lemon is also a natural skin whitener, and also helps reduce skin redness. You need to have 1 tbsp of freshly-squeezed lemon juice, cotton balls or Q-tips, and even yogurt, if you want.

Now, what you should do is rinse your face with clean water, and then pat it dry. Use Q-tips, cotton balls, or your fingers to dab into the lemon juice, and apply it to the affected areas. Use yogurt to cool it down if you feel like it stings too much for your liking.

Oatmeal

An oatmeal mask has been said to reduce redness and inflammation, and can help you feel better from the inside out. With some honey, it can be a strong acne remedy.

You will need one serving of steel-cut oatmeal—or any kind that you want, 2 tbsp raw honey, and some water. Cook oatmeal the way you normally would, and then add 2 tbsp of honey once it's done. Once it cools down considerably, apply it to your skin, and leave it there for at least 20 to 30 minutes. Rinse with warm water and pat dry.

Honey and Avocado Mask

Avocado has a good amount of nutrients that can make the skin soft and supple—and helps to combat acne. For this, you need an avocado and a tablespoon of honey.

Use water to rinse your face and then pat it dry. Take out the flesh of an avocado, mash it up, and then mix it with honey. Mash and stir until you've formed a paste out of it.

Then, apply the mixture on your skin and let it stay there for 15 to 20 minutes. Wash it off with lukewarm water afterwards, and then apply moisturizer to your skin.

Chapter 6:

Your Routine Is Key

Finally, you should keep in mind that a great routine is the ultimate key to success. By consistently keeping track of your food intake, your environment, and any natural DIY remedies you undertake, you will be able to see what works and what doesn't for your skin. Remember that everyone's skin is different and only by experimentation will you know the formula that best suits you!

Cleanse with some oil in the evening

You can normalize oil production with your face by making use of a tried and tested oil-cleaning routine that many who used to have acne—and have gotten rid of it—swear by.

What you have to do is get your oil mixture—possibly tea tree, then dilute the oil by mixing it with 9 parts water. Apply to the affected areas. You can also increase the amount, granted you're comfortable with it, apply it undiluted onto your skin.

You can then pour ½ tsp of the oil mixture to your palms, rub your hands together, and then rub them gently on your face for at least 30 seconds to 2 minutes so that the oil can easily penetrate your skin—make sure to focus on the affected areas. Wet a hand towel with below scalding water and then make sure to wring it out. Then, fold the towel so heat or steam can be kept in, and spread it over your face—don't use extremely hot water that could potentially burn you.

Use a washcloth to cover the towel so that the steam will be kept in, and then leave it on until it has cooled to room temperature. Use the washcloth to wipe your face. Repeat at least once or twice, and you'll see that oil production in your face will begin to normalize!

Scrub with sugar in the morning

Sugar isn't good to digest when you have acne, but it can be helpful when applied topically. What you can do here is mix it with olive oil or honey, or water, then scrub it on your face.

To be specific, you can use 1 ½ cups brown sugar, 1 ½ cups white sugar, 2-3 Tbsp of coarse sea salt, 1 ½ cups light or dark sugar, 10 Tbsp of pure vanilla extract, ½ cup of Extra Virgin Olive Oil, and 1 whole vanilla bean. Mix 1 ½ cups of brown and white sugar together, and add coarse sea salt—to make way for exfoliation, and then add vanilla bean, and make sure to mix well.

Put 2 cups of this salt/sugar/vanilla mixture in a measuring cup, and just pack it down until it is snug. Add the rest of the extra virgin olive oil, and allow it to soak through what you have mixed, and then add the rest of the salt/vanilla/sugar mixture.

Now, add 4 to 5 tbsp of pure vanilla, mix it all together, and spoon the scrub into your chosen containers. Use the scrub on your face like you would normal facial scrubs, leave it there for a good 10 to 15 minutes, and use lukewarm water for rinsing! This should definitely help you start your day right!

Apply honey and milk at least twice a day

For this, you'll need full-fat milk or yogurt—just at least a teaspoon, and 1 Tbsp of raw, natural honey. What you have to do now is let the milk or yogurt come to room temperature, and then mix it with 1 Tbsp of raw honey.

Use a cotton pad to apply the mixture, and then add another one—keep on adding until you feel the mixture setting on your skin. Allow it to sit for a good 10 to 15 minutes, and then use a washcloth to wash your mask off, and get rid of loosened, dead skin cells, as well!

Use Clove Acne Control

Take note that this is different from simple clove essential oil. What you can do here is buy one of those Clove Acne Control bottles, which is a proprietary blend of clove, jojoba, and other essential oils that work great on the skin.

Dab some of the oil—just a few drops—on a Q-tip or cotton ball, and dab the cotton ball or Q-tip gently on the affected areas. Do not use the whole bottle as it may be damaging to your skin!

Wash and change your pillowcases

Your pillowcases could have a lot to do with the state of your face, mostly because you spend eight hours a day rubbing your skin onto it's surface—and you get all the dirt and residue!

It's recommended that you wash your pillowcases at least once a week—twice if you can, so that all the residue won't be rubbed onto your skin and give you pimples, acne, and other skin irritations.

It might also be beneficial to go with satin pillowcases, as it is easier to clean them than other types, and can also prevent future breakouts.

Use mint to freshen your face up in the afternoon

After a long day at work or in school, your face will have probably undergone loads of stress already. Thus, it's smart to freshen up your face—and for that, you can use mint. Mint is a natural anti-inflammatory agent because it contains menthol, so it also is able to get rid of irritation and pain.
What you need to do is gather some fresh mint leaves. Then, rinse your face with clean water, and make sure to pat it dry after.

Crush the leaves thoroughly, and then use mortar and pestle or a blender to crush the leaves up. Then, once the leaves have been crushed, apply them to your face—just apply the crushed leaves together with the juice, and let it stay there for a good 5 to 10 minutes before using cold water for rinsing.

These are just some of the things you could do in your day to help yourself get rid of acne. You can also refer to chapters 5 and 6 to change the routine a bit, and make sure you try various natural remedies so you can see which works well for you. By doing so, you'll get to give your face a great new lease on life!

Chapter 7:

Acne Free Forever

Sometimes it seems as if your dream of having clear skin is impossible due to your acne problem. You have tried a lot of ways to solve this problem but trying for months and months has never brought you the results you want.

The last thing that you want in your life is a big zit on your face, but don't give up! The keys for those that have genetic pre-disposition to acne are to be as strict with these guidelines as possible. Surely, you will be able to come across an effective remedy that you can easily implement.

In conclusion, the recommended order of techniques you should follow as a newbie are:

First, take care of your hygiene. The hand-washing, body-scrubbing, and cleaning of your pores every day is the easiest to begin with and can bring you great results if you've been neglecting these in the past.

Second, make sure your diet and exercise is in check. Try to eat as many green, leafy vegetables as possible and try to flush out your pores as often as you can by drinking plenty of water each day, as well as exercising. Drink preferably around a gallon of water a day, if you'd like to measure. A daily jog will do wonders to get the sweat flowing through your pores and opening them up. After the pores open from your jog, head to the shower and scrub!

Acne does not have to ruin your life. By resorting to some simple natural ways provided in this book, you will be able to get rid of those blemishes. Now that you have gotten some tips and ideas, go fight that acne. Begin your journey towards clear skin today! It does take a lot of time and patience to finally get rid of that acne, but if you stick to the process, your goal of acne-free skin will be achieved.

Once you get rid of the acne, do what is necessary to prevent it from happening again.

That is the number one natural way to be acne-free forever.

It might be years already since you've began suffering from acne breakouts thinking that you would no longer have that flawless skin you've always wanted. However, with the right care, determination, and patience, you will surely achieve your goal.

If you aim for acne-free skin forever, living healthfully is your only choice. To get over this mental block, try to envision yourself as a "healthy and clean person". Don't take part in actions that do not bring you closer to that ultimate goal of a healthy and clean person. By viewing yourself with these attributes, you are more likely to adopt the habits and begin to turn things around.

www.ingramcontent.com/pod-product-compliance
Lightning Source LLC
Chambersburg PA
CBHW070458290526
45790CB00003B/1003